The New Mediterranean Diet Recipe Book

Get the Body You Want Without Feeling That You Are on a Diet with Foolproof, Simple and Delicious Recipes

Honey Ward

Table of Contents

INTRODUCTION..5

BREAKFAST RECIPES..9

1. Raspberries and Yogurt Smoothie....................................9

2. Homemade Muesli...10

3. Tangerine and Pomegranate Breakfast Fruit Salad 12

4. Feta Frittata...14

5. Smoked Salmon and Poached Eggs on Toast 16

6. Honey Almond Ricotta Spread with Peaches.....................18

7. Mediterranean Eggs Cups...20

8. Low-Carb Baked Eggs with Avocado and Feta 22

9. Mediterranean Eggs White Breakfast Sandwich with Roasted Tomatoes...24

10. Greek Yogurt Pancakes 26

LUNCH RECIPES...29

11. Small Pasta and Beans Pot.....................................29

12. Wild Rice, Celery, and Cauliflower Pilaf............................31

13. Minestrone Chickpeas and Macaroni Casserole.................33

14. Slow Cooked Turkey and Brown Rice....................................35

15. Papaya, Jicama, and Peas Rice Bowl 37

16. Italian Baked Beans 39

17. Cannellini Bean Lettuce Wraps...41

18. Oyster Stew..43

19. Potatoes and Lentils Stew......................................44

20. Lamb and Potatoes Stew 46

21. Ground Pork and Tomatoes Soup...47

22. Minty Lamb Stew..48

23. Peas and Orzo Soup..50

24. Turmeric Chard Soup 51

DINNER RECIPES **54**

25. Greek Meatballs 54

26. Lamb with String Beans..56

27. Greek Lamb Chop..58

28. Skillet Braised Cod with Asparagus and Potatoes 59

29. Savory Vegetable Pancakes 61

30. Mediterranean Tuna Noodle Casserole.........................63

31. Acquapazza Snapper 65

MEAT RECIPES **68**

32. Flank Steak with Orange-Herb Pistou 68

33. Braised Short Ribs with Red Wine.............................70

34. Beef Kofta 72

35. Spicy Beef with Olives and Feta................................73

36. Best Ever Beef Stew...74

37. One Pot Mediterranean Spiced Beef and Macaroni..............76

38. Beef and Cheese Gratin...78

SIDE DISH AND PIZZA **81**

39. Lemony Barley and Yogurt.......................................81

40. Chard and Couscous 82

41. Chili Cabbage and Coconut 83

42. Chickpeas, Figs and Couscous...................................84

43. Cheesy Tomato Salad...85

44. Balsamic Tomato Mix 86

VEGETARIAN DISHES..**88**

45. Steamed Squash Chowder 88

46. Steamed Zucchini-Paprika 90

47. Orange and Cucumber Salad 90

48.   Parsley and Corn Salad..92

FISH AND SEAFOOD **94**

49.   Dijon Mustard and Lime Marinated Shrimp 94

50.   Dill Relish on White Sea Bass 96

51.   Garlic Roasted Shrimp with Zucchini Pasta.........................98

APPETIZER AND SNAK RECIPES **100**

52.   Greek Fava..100

53.   Hummus, Feta & Bell Pepper Crackers 101

54.   Tomato & Basil Bruschetta 102

DESSERT RECIPES..**104**

55.   Wrapped Plums...104

56.   Marinated Feta and Artichokes...105

57.   Tuna Croquettes..106

58.   Smoked Salmon Crudités..108

59.   Citrus-Marinated Olives...109

60.   Olive Tapenade with Anchovies..110

INTRODUCTION

The traditional Mediterranean diet is described as a set of eating habits based on scientific evidence that promotes health and longevity.

Since researchers have not uniformly described Western-style eating patterns to use as a reference, it is impossible to pinpoint precisely the facets of the Mediterranean diet are advantageous. However, a substantial number of people agree that the so-called Mediterranean diet is beneficial. It's no surprise that it's linked to weight loss because of its amazingly good fats packed full of food.

Unlike other diets and fads, the Mediterranean diet's key aim is to fully turn your eating habits into one that gives you a cleaner, more healthy, and healthier version of what you enjoy. If you choose to adopt a Mediterranean diet, you should choose one that emphasizes food classes rather than individual foods.

Olives, olive oil, almonds, and seeds are some of the most essential items in the Mediterranean diet that I love (anyone on the Seattle Sutton Healthy Eating Plan will tell you that this is the right combination for a Mediterranean diet, so I'm here for you).

The Mediterranean diet is also listed as one of the balanced food programs in the American Dietary Guidelines, and the rules are somewhat close. The MIND diet is a reasonable paradigm to emulate for those with Parkinson's disease, but the general pattern of the "Mediterranean Diet" is consistent with the AHA's nutritional guidelines.

Choosing high-quality ingredients for your everyday needs is one way to alter the Mediterranean diet to better serve your interests. Since a plant-based diet is healthier for the world and the "Mediterranean diet" is more about nutrition, natural produce, it's nice that you don't have to worry about choosing fresh ingredients while cooking Mediterranean foods. The plants - the Mediterranean diet's concentrated nature makes it a very healthy diet. You've devised an excellent formula for living a healthier life, but the consistency of your fresh food must be matched with a healthy mix of grains, fruits, nuts, cereals, legumes, dairy products, eggs, fish, poultry, pork, seafood, and dairy products.

To reflect the healthier standard Mediterranean diet, the original Mediterranean diet pyramid was developed using the most up-to-date nutritional studies. In our brochure "Mediterranean Diet," we explain the Mediterranean Diet, its rules, and its advantages to help you master it.

Since the nutritional effects of the "Mediterranean diet" were found in the late 19th and early 20th centuries, the Cretan variant of the Mediterranean diet became the subject of medical studies on the "Mediterranean diet." The Mediterranean diet has made its way into medical awareness, and the nutritional effects of this diet are no longer being ignored.

There are many Mediterranean diets, as the term refers to the common foods and dietary habits of Mediterranean nations.

As a result, some Mediterranean nations, such as Greece, Italy, Spain, Cyprus, and Italy, have influenced certain sites. Then there are some regions of the world, such as the Middle East and North Africa, that inspire a particular cuisine, but there is no such thing as a "Mediterranean diet."

We may infer from this analysis that the Mediterranean diet is the safest way to live, and that a diet based on the values of the standard Mediterranean diet is linked to longer survival. The first step in beginning the "Mediterranean Diet" is to determine which diet is better for you and your health and well-being - both mentally and physically. While this does not seem like anything to dairy enthusiasts, the Mediterranean diet's main precept is to feed in moderation.

The Mediterranean diet allows you to consume foods in their most nutrient-dense shape, making it a healthy option for protein-hungry people as well as those with high blood pressure.

Unlike the paleo or keto diets, the Mediterranean diet would not entail the elimination of whole food groups like legumes and cereals or the use of fewer than 50 grams of carbohydrates a day. It is reasonably simple to obey since it does not enforce stringent calorie limits or specifically exempt foods from the diet.

Replacing refined grains with whole grains is one of the simplest Mediterranean diet measures, according to Toups. Unlike the paleo or keto diets, the Mediterranean diet does not necessitate home cooking for the majority of meals, according to the American Dietetic Association.

BREAKFAST RECIPES

1. Raspberries and Yogurt Smoothie

Preparation Time: 5 minutes

Cooking Time: 0 minutes

Servings: 2

INGREDIENTS:

- 2 cups raspberries
- ½ cup Greek yogurt
- ½ cup almond milk
- ½ tsp vanilla extract

DIRECTIONS:

1. In your blender, combine the raspberries with the milk, vanilla, and the yogurt, pulse well, divide into 2 glasses and serve for breakfast.

NUTRITION: Calories 245 Fat: 9.5g Carbs: 5.6g Protein: 1.6g

2. Homemade Muesli

Preparation Time: 15 minutes

Cooking Time: 20 minutes

Servings: 8

INGREDIENTS:

- 3 ½ cups rolled oats
- ½ cup wheat bran
- ½ tsp kosher salt
- ½ tsp ground cinnamon
- ½ cup sliced almonds
- ¼ cup raw pecans, coarsely chopped
- ¼ cup raw pepitas (shelled pumpkin seeds)
- ½ cup unsweetened coconut flakes
- ¼ cup dried apricots, coarsely chopped
- ¼ cup dried cherries

DIRECTIONS:

1. Take a medium bowl and combine the oats, wheat bran, salt, and cinnamon. Stir well. Place the mixture onto a baking sheet.
2. Next place the almonds, pecans, and pepitas onto another baking sheet and toss. Pop both trays into the oven and heat to 350°F. Bake for 10-12 minutes. Remove from the oven and pop to one side.
3. Leave the nuts to cool but take the one with the oats, sprinkle with the coconut, and pop back into the oven for 5 minutes more. Remove and leave to cool.

4. Find a large bowl and combine the contents of both trays then stir well to combine. Throw in the apricots and cherries and stir well. Pop into an airtight container until required.

NUTRITION: Calories 250 Fat: 10g Carbs: 36g Protein: 7g

3. Tangerine and Pomegranate Breakfast Fruit Salad

Preparation Time: 15 minutes

Cooking Time: 20 minutes

Servings: 5

INGREDIENTS:

- For the grains:
- 1 cup pearl or hulled barley
- 3 cups of water
- 3 tbsps. Olive oil, divided
- ½ tsp kosher salt
- For the fruit:
- ½ large pineapple, peeled and cut into 1 ½" chunks
- 6 tangerines
- 1 ¼ cups pomegranate seeds
- 1 small bunch of fresh mint
- For the dressing:
- 1/3 cup honey
- Juice and finely grated zest of 1 lemon
- Juice and finely grated zest of 2 limes
- ½ tsp kosher salt
- ¼ cup olive oil
- ¼ cup toasted hazelnut oil (olive oil is fine too)

DIRECTIONS:

1. Place the grain into a strainer and rinse well. Grab 2 baking sheets, line with paper, and add the grain. Spread well to cover then leave to dry.

2. Next, place the water into a saucepan and pop over medium heat. Place a skillet over medium heat, add 2 tbsps. Of the oil then add the barley. Toast for 2 minutes.

3. Add the water and salt and bring to a boil. Reduce to simmer and cook for 40 minutes until most of the liquid has been absorbed. Turn off the heat and leave to stand for 10 minutes to steam cook the rest.

4. Meanwhile, grab a medium bowl and add the honey, juices, zest, and salt, and stir well. Add the olive oil then nut oil and stir again. Pop until the fridge until needed.

5. Remove the lid from the barley then place it onto another prepared baking sheet and leave to cool. Drizzle with oil and leave to cool completely then pop into the fridge.

6. When ready to serve, divide the grains, pineapple, orange, pomegranate, and mint between the bowls. Drizzle with the dressing then serve and enjoy.

NUTRITION: Calories 400 Fat: 23g Carbs: 50g Protein: 3g

4. Feta Frittata

Preparation Time: 15 minutes

Cooking Time: 25 minutes

Servings: 2

Ingredients:

- 1 small clove Garlic
- 1 Green onion
- 2 Large eggs
- ½ cup Egg substitute
- 4 tbsp. Crumbled feta cheese - divided
- 1/3 cup Plum tomato
- 4 thin Avocado slices
- 2 tbsp. Reduced-fat sour cream
- Also Needed: 6-inch skillet

Directions:

1. Thinly slice/mince the onion, garlic, and tomato. Peel the avocado before slicing. Heat the pan using the medium temperature setting and spritz it with cooking oil.
2. Whisk the egg substitute, eggs, and the feta cheese. Add the egg mixture into the pan. Cover and simmer for four to six minutes.
3. Sprinkle it using the rest of the feta cheese and tomato. Cover and continue cooking until the eggs are set or about two to three more minutes.

4. Wait for about five minutes before cutting it into halves. Serve with the avocado and sour cream.

Nutrition: Calories: 460 Carbs: 8g Fat: 37g Protein: 24g

5. Smoked Salmon and Poached Eggs on Toast

Preparation Time: 10 minutes

Cooking Time: 4 minutes

Servings: 4

Ingredients:

- 2 oz avocado smashed
- 2 slices of bread toasted
- Pinch of kosher salt and cracked black pepper
- 1/4 tsp freshly squeezed lemon juice
- 2 eggs see notes, poached
- 3.5 oz smoked salmon
- 1 TBSP. thinly sliced scallions
- Splash of Kikkoman soy sauce optional
- Microgreens are optional

Directions:

1. Take a small bowl and then smash the avocado into it. Then, add the lemon juice and also a pinch of salt into the mixture. Then, mix it well and set aside.
2. After that, poach the eggs and toast the bread for some time. Once the bread is toasted, you will have to spread the avocado on both slices and after that, add the smoked salmon to each slice.
3. Thereafter, carefully transfer the poached eggs to the respective toasts. Add a splash of Kikkoman soy sauce

and some cracked pepper; then, just garnish with scallions and microgreens.

Nutrition: Calories: 459 Protein: 31 g Fat: 22 g Carbs: 33 g

6. Honey Almond Ricotta Spread with Peaches

Preparation Time: 5 minutes

Cooking Time: 8 minutes

Servings: 4

Ingredients:

- 1/2 cup Fisher Sliced Almonds
- 1 cup whole milk ricotta
- 1/4 teaspoon almond extract
- zest from an orange, optional
- 1 teaspoon honey
- hearty whole-grain toast
- English muffin or bagel
- extra Fisher sliced almonds
- sliced peaches
- extra honey for drizzling

Directions:

1. Cut peaches into a proper shape and then brush them with olive oil. After that, set it aside. Take a bowl; combine the ingredients for the filling. Set aside.

2. Then just pre-heat grill to medium. Place peaches cut side down onto the greased grill. Close lid cover and then just grill until the peaches have softened, approximately 6-10 minutes, depending on the size of the peaches.

3. Then you will have to place peach halves onto a serving plate. Put a spoon of about 1 tablespoon of ricotta mixture into the cavity (you are also allowed to use a small scooper).
4. Sprinkle it with slivered almonds, crushed amaretti cookies, and honey. Decorate with the mint leaves.

Nutrition: Calories: 187 Protein: 7 g Fat: 9 g Carbs: 18 g

7. Mediterranean Eggs Cups

Preparation Time: 10 minutes

Cooking Time: 20 minutes

Servings: 8

Ingredients:

- 1 cup spinach, finely diced
- 1/2 yellow onion, finely diced
- 1/2 cup sliced sun-dried tomatoes
- 4 large basil leaves, finely diced
- Pepper and salt to taste
- 1/3 cup feta cheese crumbles
- 8 large eggs
- 1/4 cup milk (any kind)

Directions:

1. Warm the oven to 375°F. Then, roll the dough sheet into a 12x8-inch rectangle. Then, cut in half lengthwise.
2. After that, you will have to cut each half crosswise into 4 pieces, forming 8 (4x3-inch) pieces dough. Then, press each into the bottom and up sides of the ungreased muffin cup.
3. Trim dough to keep the dough from touching, if essential. Set aside. Then, you will have to combine the eggs, salt, pepper in the bowl and beat it with a whisk until well mixed. Set aside.

4. Melt the butter in 12-inch skillet over medium heat until sizzling; add bell peppers. You will have to cook it, stirring occasionally, 2-3 minutes or until crisply tender.

5. After that, add spinach leaves; continue cooking until spinach is wilted. Then just add egg mixture and prosciutto.

6. Divide the mixture evenly among prepared muffin cups. Finally, bake it for 14-17 minutes or until the crust is golden brown.

Nutrition: Calories: 240 Protein: 9 g Fat: 16 g Carbs: 13 g

8. Low-Carb Baked Eggs with Avocado and Feta

Preparation Time: 10 minutes

Cooking Time: 15 minutes

Servings: 2

Ingredients:

- 1 avocado
- 4 eggs
- 2-3 tbsp. crumbled feta cheese
- Nonstick cooking spray
- Pepper and salt to taste

Directions:

1. First, you will have to preheat the oven to 400 degrees f. After that, when the oven is on the proper temperature, you will have to put the gratin dishes right on the baking sheet.
2. Then, leave the dishes to heat in the oven for almost 10 minutes After that process, you need to break the eggs into individual ramekins.
3. Then, let the avocado and eggs come to room temperature for at least 10 minutes. Then, peel the avocado properly and cut it each half into 6-8 slices.
4. You will have to remove the dishes from the oven and spray them with the non-stick spray. Then, you will have to arrange all the sliced avocados in the dishes

and tip two eggs into each dish. Sprinkle with feta, add pepper and salt to taste, serve.

Nutrition: Calories: 280 Protein: 11 g Fat: 23 g Carbs: 10 g

9. Mediterranean Eggs White Breakfast Sandwich with Roasted Tomatoes

Preparation Time: 15 minutes

Cooking Time: 10 minutes

Servings: 2

Ingredients:

- Salt and pepper to taste
- ¼ cup egg whites
- 1 teaspoon chopped fresh herbs like rosemary, basil, parsley,
- 1 whole-grain seeded ciabatta roll
- 1 teaspoon butter
- 1-2 slices Muenster cheese
- 1 tablespoon pesto
- About ½ cup roasted tomatoes
- 10 ounces grape tomatoes
- 1 tablespoon extra-virgin olive oil
- Black pepper and salt to taste

Directions:

1. First, you will have to melt the butter over medium heat in the small nonstick skillet. Then, mix the egg whites with pepper and salt.
2. Then, sprinkle it with the fresh herbs. After that cook it for almost 3-4 minutes or until the eggs are done, then flip it carefully.

3. Meanwhile, toast ciabatta bread in the toaster. Place the egg on the bottom half of the sandwich rolls, then top with cheese
4. Add roasted tomatoes and the top half of roll. To make a roasted tomato, preheat the oven to 400 degrees. Then, slice the tomatoes in half lengthwise.
5. Place on the baking sheet and drizzle with olive oil. Season it with pepper and salt and then roast in the oven for about 20 minutes. Skins will appear wrinkled when done.

Nutrition: Calories: 458 Protein: 21 g Fat: 24 g Carbs: 51 g

10. Greek Yogurt Pancakes

Preparation Time: 10 minutes

Cooking Time: 5 minutes

Servings: 2

Ingredients:

- 1 cup all-purpose flour
- 1 cup whole-wheat flour
- 1/4 teaspoon salt
- 4 teaspoons baking powder
- 1 tablespoon sugar
- 1 1/2 cups unsweetened almond milk
- 2 teaspoons vanilla extract
- 2 large eggs
- 1/2 cup plain 2% Greek yogurt
- Fruit, for serving
- Maple syrup, for serving

Directions:

1. First, you will have to pour the curds into the bowl and mix them well until creamy. After that, you will have to add egg whites and mix them well until combined.
2. Then take a separate bowl, pour the wet mixture into the dry mixture. Stir to combine. The batter will be extremely thick.

3. Then, simply spoon the batter onto the sprayed pan heated too medium-high. The batter must make 4 large pancakes.
4. Then, you will have to flip the pancakes once when they start to bubble a bit on the surface. Cook until golden brown on both sides.

Nutrition: Calories: 166 Protein: 14 g Fat: 5 g Carbs: 52g

LUNCH RECIPES

11. Small Pasta and Beans Pot

Preparation time: 15 minutes

Cooking time: 15 minutes

Servings: 2-4

INGREDIENTS:

- 1 pound (454 g) small whole wheat pasta
- 1 (14.5-ounce / 411-g) can diced tomatoes, juice reserved
- 1 (15-ounce / 425-g) can cannellini beans, drained and rinsed
- 2 tablespoons no-salt-added tomato paste
- 1 red or yellow bell pepper, chopped
- 1 yellow onion, chopped
- 1 tablespoon Italian seasoning mix
- 3 garlic cloves, minced
- ¼ teaspoon crushed red pepper flakes, optional
- 1 tablespoon extra-virgin olive oil
- 5 cups water
- 1 bunch kale, stemmed and chopped
- ½ cup pitted Kalamata olives, chopped
- 1 cup sliced basil

DIRECTIONS:

1. Except for the kale, olives, and basil, combine all the ingredients in a pot. Stir to mix well. Bring to a boil over high heat. Stir constantly.
2. Reduce the heat to medium high and add the kale. Cook for 10 minutes or until the pasta is al dente. Stir constantly. Transfer all of them on a large plate and serve with olives and basil on top.

NUTRITION: Calories: 357 Fat: 7.6g Protein: 18.2g Carbs: 64.5g

12. Wild Rice, Celery, and Cauliflower Pilaf

Preparation time: 15 minutes

Cooking time: 45 minutes

Servings: 4

INGREDIENTS:

- 1 tablespoon olive oil, plus more for greasing the baking dish
- 1 cup wild rice
- 2 cups low-sodium chicken broth
- 1 sweet onion, chopped
- 2 stalks celery, chopped
- 1 teaspoon minced garlic
- 2 carrots, peeled, halved lengthwise, and sliced
- ½ cauliflower head, cut into small florets
- 1 teaspoon chopped fresh thyme
- Sea salt, to taste

DIRECTIONS:

1. Preheat the oven to 350ºf (180ºc). Line a baking sheet with parchment paper and grease with olive oil.
2. Put the wild rice in a saucepan, then pour in the chicken broth. Bring to a boil. Reduce the heat to low and simmer for 30 minutes or until the rice is plump.
3. Meanwhile, heat the remaining olive oil in an oven-proof skillet over medium-high heat until shimmering.

4. Add the onion, celery, and garlic to the skillet and sauté for 3 minutes or until the onion is translucent.

5. Add the carrots and cauliflower to the skillet and sauté for 5 minutes. Turn off the heat and set aside.

6. Pour the cooked rice in the skillet with the vegetables. Sprinkle with thyme and salt. Set the skillet in the preheated oven and bake for 15 minutes or until the vegetables are soft. Serve immediately.

NUTRITION: Calories: 214 Fat: 3.9g Protein: 7.2g Carbs: 37.9g

13. Minestrone Chickpeas and Macaroni Casserole

Preparation time: 15 minutes

Cooking time: 7 hours & 25 minutes

Servings: 5

INGREDIENTS:

- 1 (15-ounce / 425-g) can chickpeas, drained and rinsed
- 1 (28-ounce / 794-g) can diced tomatoes, with the juice
- 1 (6-ounce / 170-g) can no-salt-added tomato paste
- 3 medium carrots, sliced
- 3 cloves garlic, minced
- 1 medium yellow onion, chopped
- 1 cup low-sodium vegetable soup
- ½ teaspoon dried rosemary
- 1 teaspoon dried oregano
- 2 teaspoons maple syrup
- ½ teaspoon sea salt
- ¼ teaspoon ground black pepper
- ½ pound (227-g) fresh green beans, trimmed and cut into bite-size pieces
- 1 cup macaroni pasta
- 2 ounces (57 g) Parmesan cheese, grated

DIRECTIONS:

1. Except for the green beans, pasta, and Parmesan cheese, combine all the ingredients in the slow cooker and stir

to mix well. Put the slow cooker lid on and cook on low for 7 hours.

2. Fold in the pasta and green beans. Put the lid on and cook on high for 20 minutes or until the vegetable are soft and the pasta is al dente.

3. Pour them in a large serving bowl and spread with Parmesan cheese before serving.

NUTRITION: Calories: 349 Fat: 6.7g Protein: 16.5g Carbs: 59.9g

14. Slow Cooked Turkey and Brown Rice

Preparation time: 15 minutes

Cooking time: 3 hours & 10 minutes

Servings: 6

INGREDIENTS:

- 1 tablespoon extra-virgin olive oil
- 1½ pounds (680 g) ground turkey
- 2 tablespoons chopped fresh sage, divided
- 2 tablespoons chopped fresh thyme, divided
- 1 teaspoon sea salt
- ½ teaspoon ground black pepper
- 2 cups brown rice
- 1 (14-ounce / 397-g) can stewed tomatoes, with the juice
- ¼ cup pitted and sliced Kalamata olives
- 3 medium zucchinis, sliced thinly
- ¼ cup chopped fresh flat-leaf parsley
- 1 medium yellow onion, chopped
- 1 tablespoon plus 1 teaspoon balsamic vinegar
- 2 cups low-sodium chicken stock
- 2 garlic cloves, minced
- ½ cup grated Parmesan cheese, for serving

DIRECTIONS:

1. Heat the olive oil in a nonstick skillet over medium-high heat until shimmering. Add the ground turkey and sprinkle with 1 tablespoon of sage, 1 tablespoon of thyme, salt and ground black pepper.

2. Sauté for 10 minutes or until the ground turkey is lightly browned. Pour them in the slow cooker, then pour in the remaining ingredients, except for the Parmesan. Stir to mix well.

3. Put the lid on and cook on high for 3 hours or until the rice and vegetables are tender. Pour them in a large serving bowl, then spread with Parmesan cheese before serving.

NUTRITION: Calories: 499 Fat: 16.4g Protein: 32.4g Carbs: 56.5g

15. Papaya, Jicama, and Peas Rice Bowl

Preparation time: 15 minutes

Cooking time: 45 minutes

Servings: 4

INGREDIENTS:

- Sauce:
- Juice of ¼ lemon
- 2 teaspoons chopped fresh basil
- 1 tablespoon raw honey
- 1 tablespoon extra-virgin olive oil
- Sea salt, to taste
- Rice:
- 1½ cups wild rice
- 2 papayas, peeled, seeded, and diced
- 1 jicama, peeled and shredded
- 1 cup snow peas, julienned
- 2 cups shredded cabbage
- 1 scallion, white and green parts, chopped

DIRECTIONS:

1. Combine the ingredients for the sauce in a bowl. Stir to mix well. Set aside until ready to use. Pour the wild rice in a saucepan, then pour in enough water to cover. Bring to a boil.
2. Reduce the heat to low, then simmer for 45 minutes or until the wild rice is soft and plump. Drain and transfer to a large serving bowl.

3. Top the rice with papayas, jicama, peas, cabbage, and scallion. Pour the sauce over and stir to mix well before serving.

NUTRITION: Calories: 446 Fat: 7.9g Protein: 13.1g Carbs: 85.8g

16. Italian Baked Beans

Preparation time: 5 minutes

Cooking time: 15 minutes

Servings: 6

INGREDIENTS:

- 2 teaspoons extra-virgin olive oil
- ½ cup minced onion (about ¼ onion)
- 1 (12-ounce) can low-sodium tomato paste
- ¼ cup red wine vinegar
- 2 tablespoons honey
- ¼ teaspoon ground cinnamon
- ½ cup water
- 2 (15-ounce) cans cannellini or great northern beans, undrained

DIRECTIONS:

1. In a medium saucepan over medium heat, heat the oil. Add the onion and cook for 5 minutes, stirring frequently.
2. Add the tomato paste, vinegar, honey, cinnamon, and water, and mix well. Turn the heat to low. Drain and rinse one can of the beans in a colander and add to the saucepan.
3. Pour the entire second can of beans (including the liquid) into the saucepan. Let it cook for 10 minutes, stirring occasionally, and serve.

4. Ingredient tip: Switch up this recipe by making new variations of the homemade ketchup. Instead of the cinnamon, try ¼ teaspoon of smoked paprika and 1 tablespoon of hot sauce. Serve.

NUTRITION: Calories: 236 Fat: 3g Carbohydrates: 42g Protein: 10g

17. Cannellini Bean Lettuce Wraps

Preparation time: 15 minutes

Cooking time: 10 minutes

Servings: 4

INGREDIENTS:

- 1 tablespoon extra-virgin olive oil
- ½ cup diced red onion (about ¼ onion)
- ¾ cup chopped fresh tomatoes (about 1 medium tomato)
- ¼ teaspoon freshly ground black pepper
- 1 (15-ounce) can cannellini or great northern beans, drained and rinsed
- ¼ cup finely chopped fresh curly parsley
- ½ cup Lemony Garlic Hummus or ½ cup prepared hummus
- 8 romaine lettuce leaves

DIRECTIONS:

1. In a large skillet over medium heat, heat the oil. Add the onion and cook for 3 minutes, stirring occasionally.
2. Add the tomatoes and pepper and cook for 3 more minutes, stirring occasionally. Add the beans and cook for 3 more minutes, stirring occasionally. Remove from the heat, and mix in the parsley.
3. Spread 1 tablespoon of hummus over each lettuce leaf. Evenly spread the warm bean mixture down the center of each leaf.

4. Fold one side of the lettuce leaf over the filling lengthwise, then fold over the other side to make a wrap and serve.

NUTRITION: Calories: 211 Fat: 8g Carbohydrates: 28g Protein: 10g

18. Oyster Stew

Preparation time: 10 minutes

Cooking time: 1 hour and 10 minutes

Servings: 6

Ingredients:

- 2 garlic cloves, minced
- ¼ cup jarred roasted red peppers
- 2 teaspoons oregano, chopped
- 1-pound lamb meat, ground
- 1 tablespoon red wine vinegar
- Salt and black pepper to the taste
- 1 teaspoon red pepper flakes
- 2 tablespoons olive oil
- 1 and ½ cups chicken stock
- 36 oysters, shucked
- 1 and ½ cups canned black eyed peas, drained

Directions:

1. Heat up a pot with the oil over medium heat, add the meat and the garlic and brown for 5 minutes.
2. Add the peppers and the rest of the ingredients, bring to a simmer and cook for 15 minutes.
3. Divide the stew into bowls and serve.

Nutrition: calories 264, fat 9.3, fiber 1.2, carbs 2.3, protein 1.2

19. Potatoes and Lentils Stew

Preparation time: 10 minutes

Cooking time: 35 minutes

Servings: 4

Ingredients:

- 4 cups water
- 1 cup carrots, sliced
- 1 yellow onion, chopped
- 1 tablespoon olive oil
- 1 cup celery, chopped
- 2 garlic cloves, minced
- 2 pounds gold potatoes, cubed
- 1 and ½ cup lentils, dried
- ½ teaspoon smoked paprika
- ½ teaspoon oregano, dried
- Salt and black pepper to the taste
- 14 ounces canned tomatoes, chopped
- ½ cup cilantro, chopped

Directions:

1. Heat up a pot with the oil over medium- high heat, add the onion, garlic, celery and carrots, stir and cook for 5 minutes.
2. Add the rest of the ingredients except the cilantro, stir, bring to a simmer and cook over medium heat for 25 minutes.
3. Add the cilantro, divide the stew into bowls and serve.

Nutrition: calories 325, fat 17.3, fiber 6.8, carbs 26.4, protein 16.4

20. Lamb and Potatoes Stew

Preparation time: 10 minutes

Cooking time: 1 hour and 20 minutes

Servings: 4

Ingredients:

- 2 pounds lamb shoulder, boneless and cubed
- Salt and black pepper to the taste
- 1 yellow onion, chopped
- 3 tablespoons olive oil
- 3 tomatoes, grated
- 2 cups chicken stock
- 2 and ½ pounds gold potatoes, cubed
- ¾ cup green olives, pitted and sliced
- 1 tablespoon cilantro, chopped

Directions:

1. Heat up a pot with the oil over medium-high heat, add the lamb, and brown for 5 minutes on each side.
2. Add the onion and sauté for 5 minutes more.
3. Add the rest of the ingredients, bring to a simmer and cook over medium heat and cook for 1 hour and 10 minutes.
4. Divide the stew into bowls and serve.

Nutrition: calories 411, fat 17.4, fiber 8.4, carbs 25.5, protein 34.3

21. Ground Pork and Tomatoes Soup

Preparation time: 10 minutes

Cooking time: 40 minutes

Servings: 4

Ingredients:

- 1-pound pork meat, ground
- Salt and black pepper to the taste
- 2 garlic cloves, minced
- 2 teaspoons thyme, dried
- 2 tablespoons olive oil
- 4 cups beef stock
- A pinch of saffron powder
- 15 ounces canned tomatoes, crushed
- 1 tablespoons parsley, chopped

Directions:

1. Heat up a pot with the oil over medium heat, add the meat and the garlic and brown for 5 minutes.
2. Add the rest of the ingredients except the parsley, bring to a simmer and cook for 25 minutes.
3. Divide the soup into bowls, sprinkle the parsley on top and serve.

Nutrition: calories 372, fat 17.3, fiber 5.5, carbs 28.4, protein 17.4

22. Minty Lamb Stew

Preparation time: 10 minutes

Cooking time: 1 hour and 45 minutes

Servings: 4

Ingredients:

- 3 cups orange juice
- ½ cup mint, chopped
- Salt and black pepper to the taste
- 2 pounds lamb shoulder, boneless and cubed
- 3 tablespoons olive oil
- 1 carrot, chopped
- 1 yellow onion, chopped
- 1 celery rib, chopped
- 1 tablespoon ginger, grated
- 28 ounces canned tomatoes, crushed
- 1 tablespoon garlic, minced
- 1 cup apricots, dried and halved
- ½ cup mint, chopped
- 15 ounces canned chickpeas, drained
- 6 tablespoons Greek yogurt

Directions:

1. Heat up a pot with 2 tablespoons oil over medium-high heat, add the meat and brown for 5 minutes.
2. Add the carrot, onion, celery, garlic and the ginger, stir and sauté for 5 minutes more.

3. Add the rest of the ingredients except the yogurt, bring to a simmer and cook over medium heat for 1 hour and 30 minutes.
4. Divide the stew into bowls, top each serving with the yogurt and serve.

Nutrition: calories 355, fat 14.3, fiber 6.7, carbs 22.6, protein 15.4

23. Peas and Orzo Soup

Preparation time: 10 minutes

Cooking time: 10 minutes

Servings: 4

Ingredients:

- ½ cup orzo
- 6 cups chicken soup
- 1 and ½ cups cheddar, shredded
- Salt and black pepper to the taste
- 2 teaspoons oregano, dried
- ¼ cup yellow onion, chopped
- 3 cups baby spinach
- 2 tablespoons lime juice
- ½ cup peas

Directions:

1. Heat up a pot with the soup over medium heat, add the orzo and the rest of the ingredients except the cheese, bring to a simmer and cook for 10 minutes.
2. Add the cheese, stir, divide into bowls and serve.

Nutrition: calories 360, fat 10.2, fiber 4.7, carbs 43.3, protein 22.3

24. Turmeric Chard Soup

Preparation time: 10 minutes

Cooking time: 40 minutes

Servings: 6

Ingredients:

- 2 tablespoons olive oil
- 1-pound chard, chopped
- 1 teaspoon coriander seeds, ground
- 2 teaspoons mustard seeds
- 2 teaspoons garlic, minced
- 1 tablespoon ginger, grated
- ¼ teaspoon cardamom, ground
- ¼ teaspoon turmeric powder
- 1 yellow onion, chopped
- ¾ cup rhubarb, sliced
- Salt and black pepper to the taste
- 5 cups water
- 3 tablespoons cilantro, chopped
- 6 tablespoons yogurt

Directions:

1. Heat up a pan with the oil over medium heat, add the coriander, mustard seeds, garlic, ginger, cardamom, turmeric and the onion, stir and sauté for 5 minutes.
2. Add the rest of the ingredients except the cilantro and the yogurt, bring to a simmer and cook for 20 minutes.

3. Divide the soup into bowls, top each serving with cilantro and yogurt and serve.

Nutrition: calories 189, fat 8.3, fiber 3.4, carbs 11.7, protein 4.5

DINNER RECIPES

25. Greek Meatballs

Preparation Time: 20 minutes

Cooking Time: 25 minutes

Serving: 4

Ingredients:

- 2 whole-wheat bread slices
- 1¼ pounds ground turkey
- 1 egg
- ¼ cup seasoned whole-wheat bread crumbs
- 3 garlic cloves, minced
- ¼ red onion, grated
- ¼ cup chopped fresh Italian parsley leaves
- 2 tablespoons chopped fresh mint leaves
- 2 tablespoons chopped fresh oregano leaves
- ½ teaspoon sea salt
- ¼ teaspoon freshly ground black pepper

Direction:

1. Preheat the oven to 350°F.
2. Prep baking sheet with foil.
3. Run the bread under water to wet it, and squeeze out any excess. Rip the wet bread into small pieces and put it in a medium bowl.

4. Add the turkey, egg, bread crumbs, garlic, red onion, parsley, mint, oregano, sea salt, and pepper. Mix well. Form the mixture into ¼-cup-size balls. Place the meatballs on the prepared sheet and bake for about 25 minutes

Nutrition: 350 Calories 42g Protein 18g Fat

26. Lamb with String Beans

Preparation Time: 10 minutes

Cooking Time: 1 hour

Serving: 6

Ingredients:

- ¼ cup extra-virgin olive oil
- 6 lamb chops
- 1 teaspoon sea salt
- ½ teaspoon black pepper
- 2 tablespoons tomato paste
- 1½ cups hot water
- 1-pound green beans
- 1 onion
- 2 tomatoes

Direction:

1. In a skillet at medium-high heat, pour 2 tablespoons of olive oil.
2. Season the lamb chops with ½ teaspoon of sea salt and 1/8 teaspoon of pepper. Cook the lamb in the hot oil for about 4 minutes. Transfer the meat to a platter and set aside.
3. Put back to the heat then put the 2 tablespoons of olive oil. Heat until it shimmers.
4. Blend tomato paste in the hot water. Mix to the hot skillet along with the green beans, onion, tomatoes, and

the remaining ½ teaspoon of sea salt and ¼ teaspoon of pepper. Bring to a simmer.

5. Return the lamb chops to the pan. Boil and adjust the heat to medium-low. Simmer for 45 minutes, adding additional water as needed to adjust the thickness of the sauce.

Nutrition: 439 Calories 50g Protein 22g Fat

27. Greek Lamb Chop

Preparation Time: 10 minutes

Cooking Time: 8 minutes

Serving: 8

Ingredients:

- 8 trimmed lamb loin chops
- 2 tbsp lemon juice
- 1 tbsp dried oregano
- 1 tbsp minced garlic
- ½ tsp salt
- ¼ tsp black pepper

Direction:

1. Preheat the broiler
2. Combine oregano, garlic, lemon juice, salt and pepper and rub on both sides of the lamb. Situate lamb on a broiler pan coated with cooking spray and cook for 4 min on each side.

Nutrition: 457 Calories 49g Protein 20g Fat

28. Skillet Braised Cod with Asparagus and Potatoes

Preparation Time: 20 minutes

Cooking Time: 20 minutes

Serving: 4

Ingredients:

- 4 skinless cod fillets
- 1-pound asparagus
- 12 oz halved small purple potatoes
- Finely grated zest of ½ lemon
- Juice of ½ lemon
- ½ cup white wine
- ¼ cup torn fresh basil leaves
- 1 ½ tbsp olive oil
- 1 tbsp capers
- 3 cloves sliced garlic

Direction:

1. Take a large and tall pan on the sides and heat the oil over medium-high.
2. Season the cod abundantly with salt and pepper and put in the pan, with the hot oil, for 1 min. Carefully flip for 1 more min and after transferring the cod to a plate. Set aside.
3. Add the lemon zest, capers and garlic to the pan and mix to coat with the remaining oil in the pan and cook about 1 min. Add the wine and deglaze the

pan. Add lemon juice, potatoes, ½ tsp salt, ¼ tsp pepper and 2 cups of water and boil, adjust heat and simmer until potatoes are tender, for 10 to 12 min.

4. Mix the asparagus and cook for 2 min. Bring back the cod filets and any juices accumulated in the pan. Cook until the asparagus are tender, for about 3 min.

5. Divide the cod fillets into shallow bowls and add the potatoes and asparagus. Mix the basil in the broth left in the pan and pour over the cod.

Nutrition: 461 Calories 40g Protein 16g Fat

29. Savory Vegetable Pancakes

Preparation Time: 10 minutes

Cooking Time: 40 minutes

Serving: 7

Ingredients:

- 8 peeled carrots
- 2 cloves garlic
- 1 zucchini
- 1 bunch green onions
- ½ bunch parsley
- 1 recipe pancake batter

Direction:

1. Grate chop the zucchini and carrots using grater. Finely chop the onions, mince the garlic and roughly chop the parsley.

2. Prepare pancakes with your favorite recipe or buy them in the store, but use ¼ cup of liquid less than required, zucchini will add a large amount of liquid to the mix. Fold the vegetables in the prepared pancake batter.

3. Heat a pan over medium-high heat and brush it mildly with olive oil. With a 1/3 measuring cup to scoop the batter on the heated pan. Cook 3 to 4 min, until the outer edge has set, then turn over. Cook for another 2 min and remove from the heat.

4. Season the pancakes with plenty of salt. Serve.

Nutrition: 291 Calories 24g Protein 10g Fat

30. Mediterranean Tuna Noodle Casserole

Preparation Time: 15 minutes

Cooking Time: 40 minutes

Serving: 5

Ingredients:

- 10 oz dried egg noodles
- 9 oz halved frozen artichoke hearts
- 6 oz drained olive oil packed tuna
- 4 sliced scallions
- 1-pound sliced ¼ inch thick small red potatoes
- 2 cup milk
- ¾ cup finely grated Parmesan cheese
- ¾ cup drained capers
- ½ cup finely chopped flat-leaf parsley
- ½ cup sliced black olives
- ¼ cup flour
- 4 tbsp unsalted butter
- 2 tsp *Kosher salt, divided*

Direction:

1. Place a grill in the middle of the oven and heat to 400° F. Lightly coat a 2-quart baking tray with oil. Set aside.

2. Using a big pan of salt water to a boil. Stir in noodles and cook for 2 min less than recommended in the package directions. Strain noodles. Season

immediately with olive oil so that they don't pile up. Set aside.

3.	Fill the pan with water again and boil. Stir in potato slices and cook for 4 min. Drain well, then bring them back to the pan.

4.	Cook butter in a saucepan at medium heat, while the noodles and potatoes are cooking. When it melts and expands, add the flour and cook for about 5 min mixing constantly, until the sauce thickens slightly, about 5 min. Add 1 tsp salt and pepper to taste.

5.	Add the egg noodles to the potato pan, then pour the sauce over it. Add and mix the remaining 1 tsp of salt, capers, olive oil, tuna, artichoke hearts, shallots, parsley and ½ cup of Parmesan. Season well.

6.	Transfer to the baking tray and distribute it in a uniform layer. Season with the remaining ¼ cup of Parmesan and bake, uncovered, about 25 min.

Nutrition: 457 Calories 37g Protein 21g Fat

31. Acquapazza Snapper

Preparation Time: 10 minutes

Cooking Time: 35 minutes

Serving: 4

Ingredients:

- 1 ½ pounds cut into 4 pieces red snapper fillets
- 1 ½ coarsely chopped ripe tomatoes
- 3 cups water
- 2 tbsp olive oil
- 1 tbsp chopped thyme leaves
- 1 tbsp chopped oregano leaves
- ¼ tsp red pepper flakes
- 3 cloves minced garlic

Direction:

1. Cook oil in a casserole large enough to hold all 4 pieces of snapper fillets in a single layer over medium heat. Cook garlic and red pepper flakes
2. Add the water, tomatoes, thyme, oregano and simmer. Cover, reduce over medium-low heat and simmer for 15 min. Remove the lid and continue to simmer for another 10 min so that the liquid decreases slightly, pressing occasionally on the tomatoes. Taste and season with salt as needed.
3. Put the snapper fillets in the casserole with the skin facing down, if there is skin. Sprinkle with salt, and cook for 9 min.

4. Place the snapper fillets on 4 large, shallow bowls and put the broth around it. Serve immediately.

Nutrition: 501 Calories 52g Protein 26g Fat

MEAT RECIPES

32. Flank Steak with Orange-Herb Pistou

Preparation Time: 10 minutes

Cooking Time: 20 minutes

Servings: 4

Ingredients:

- 1-pound flank steak
- 8 tablespoons extra-virgin olive oil, divided
- 2 teaspoons salt, divided
- 1 teaspoon freshly ground black pepper, divided
- ½ cup chopped fresh flat-leaf Italian parsley
- ¼ cup chopped fresh mint leaves
- 2 garlic cloves, roughly chopped
- Zest and juice of 1 orange or 2 clementines
- 1 teaspoon red pepper flakes (optional)
- 1 tablespoon red wine vinegar

DirectionS:

1. Heat the grill to medium-high heat or, if using an oven, preheat to 400°F.

2. Rub the steak with 2 tablespoons olive oil and sprinkle with 1 teaspoon salt and ½ teaspoon pepper. Let sit at room temperature while you make the pistou.

3. In a food processor, combine the parsley, mint, garlic, orange zest and juice, remaining 1 teaspoon salt, red pepper flakes (if using), and remaining ½ teaspoon pepper. Pulse until finely chopped. With the processor running, stream in the red wine vinegar and remaining 6 tablespoons olive oil until well combined. This pistou will be more oil-based than traditional basil pesto.

4. Cook the steak on the grill, 6 to 8 minutes per side. Remove from the grill and allow to rest for 10 minutes on a cutting board. If cooking in the oven, heat a large oven-safe skillet (cast iron works great) over high heat. Add the steak and seer, 1 to 2 minutes per side, until browned. Transfer the skillet to the oven and cook 10 to 12 minutes, or until the steak reaches your desired temperature.

5. To serve, slice the steak and drizzle with the pistou.

Nutrition: Calories: 441 Total Fat: 36g Total Carbs: 3g Net Carbs: 3g Fiber: 0g Protein: 25g Sodium: 1237mg

33. Braised Short Ribs with Red Wine

Preparation Time: 10 minutes

Cooking Time: 2 minutes

Servings: 4

Ingredients:

- 1½ pounds boneless beef short ribs (if using bone-in, use 3½ pounds)
- 1 teaspoon salt
- ½ teaspoon freshly ground black pepper
- ½ teaspoon garlic powder
- ¼ cup extra-virgin olive oil
- 1 cup dry red wine (such as cabernet sauvignon or merlot)
- 2 to 3 cups beef broth, divided
- 4 sprigs rosemary

Directions:

1. Preheat the oven to 350°F.
2. Season the short ribs with salt, pepper, and garlic powder. Let sit for 10 minutes.
3. In a Dutch oven or oven-safe deep skillet, heat the olive oil over medium-high heat.
4. When the oil is very hot, add the short ribs and brown until dark in color, 2 to 3 minutes per side. Remove the meat from the oil and keep warm.
5. Add the red wine and 2 cups beef broth to the Dutch oven, whisk together, and bring to a boil. Reduce the

heat to low and simmer until the liquid is reduced to about 2 cups, about 10 minutes.

6. Return the short ribs to the liquid, which should come about halfway up the meat, adding up to 1 cup of remaining broth if needed. Cover and braise until the meat are very tender, about 1½ to 2 hours.

7. Remove from the oven and let sit, covered, for 10 minutes before serving. Serve warm, drizzled with cooking liquid.

Nutrition: Calories: 792 Total Fat: 76g Total Carbs: 2g Net Carbs: 2g Fiber: 0g Protein: 25g Sodium: 783mg

34. **Beef Kofta**

Preparation Time: 10 minutes

Cooking Time: 15 minutes

Servings: 4

Ingredients:

- 1 lb. ground beef
- 1/2 cup minced onions
- 1 tablespoon olive oil
- 1/2 teaspoon salt
- 1/2 teaspoon ground coriander
- 1/2 teaspoon ground cumin
- 1/4 teaspoon ground cinnamon
- 1/4 teaspoon allspice
- 1/4 teaspoon dried mint leaves

Directions:

1. Grab a large bowl and add all the ingredients.
2. Stir well to combine then use your hands to shape into ovals or balls.
3. Carefully thread onto skewers then brush with oil.
4. Pop into the grill and cook uncovered for 15 minutes, turning often.
5. Serve and enjoy.

Nutrition: Calories: 216 Net carbs: 4g Fat: 19g Protein: 25g

35. Spicy Beef with Olives and Feta

Preparation Time: 3 hours

Cooking Time: 6 hours

Servings: 6-8

Ingredients:

- 2 lb. stewing beef, cut into ½" pieces
- 2 x 15 oz. cans chili-seasoned diced tomatoes, undrained
- 1 cup assorted olives, pitted and halved
- 1/2 teaspoon salt
- 1/4 teaspoon pepper
- 2 cups cooked basmati rice
- 1/2 cup crumbled feta cheese

Directions:

1. Open the lid of your slow cooker and add the beef, tomatoes and olives. Stir well.
2. Cover and cook on high for 5-6 hours or low for 8-9 ours until tender.
3. Season well then serve with the rice and feta cheese.
4. Serve and enjoy.

Nutrition: Calories: 380 Net carbs: 14g Fat: 19g Protein: 36g

36. Best Ever Beef Stew

Preparation Time: 1 hour

Cooking Time: 2 hours

Servings: 6

Ingredients:

- 2 tablespoons olive oil
- 1 1/3 lb. extra- lean diced beef
- 1 large onion, sliced
- 1½ tablespoons chopped rosemary
- 5 garlic cloves, sliced
- 2/3 cup red wine (or extra stock)
- 1 2/3 cup beef stock
- 1 x 14 oz. can cherry tomatoes
- 3 mixed peppers, deseeded and thickly sliced
- 2 x 14 oz. can butterbeans, rinsed and drained
- 1 x 2.4 oz. pouch pitted Kalamata olives
- 2 tablespoons corn flour

Directions:

1. Preheat the oven to 280°F.
2. Place a Dutch oven over a medium heat and add 1 tablespoon oil.
3. Place the beef onto a flat surface, season well and cook in two batches.
4. Remove and place onto a plate when cooked.
5. Add the remaining oil and cook the onion, rosemary and garlic for 5 minutes until soft.

6. Add a pinch of salt then pour in the wine, scraping and browned bits from the pan.
7. Add the beef stock, tomatoes and peppers, stir well.
8. Add the beef, cover and bring to a simmer.
9. Pop into the oven and leave to cook for 2 hours.
10. Add the butterbeans and olive and pop back into the oven for 30 minutes.
11. Find a small bowl and combine the corn starch with a little water.
12. Pour gently into the stew, stir well and simmer until thickened.
13. Serve and enjoy.

Nutrition: Calories: 337 Net carbs: 15g Fat: 10g Protein: 31g

37. One Pot Mediterranean Spiced Beef and Macaroni

Preparation Time: 25 minutes

Cooking Time: 10 minutes

Servings: 4

INGREDIENTS:

- 2 tablespoons olive oil
- 1 lb. ground beef
- 1 cup onion, diced
- 3 cloves garlic minced
- 1 teaspoon ground cinnamon
- ½ teaspoon kosher salt
- ¼ teaspoon cayenne pepper
- ¼ teaspoon ground cloves
- ½ cup red wine
- 2 Roma tomatoes diced
- 8 oz. can tomato sauce
- 2 cups macaroni or cavatappi noodles
- 2 cups beef broth
- ¼ cup parmesan cheese, grated

Directions:

1.   Place a large pan over a medium heat and add the olive oil.

2.   Add the beef, onion and garlic and cook for 10 minutes or so until soft.

3. Drain away the remaining grease then add the cinnamon, cayenne and cloves.
4. Cook for 3-4 minutes then add the red wine, tomatoes and tomato sauce.
5. Simmer for 5 minutes then add the noodles and the broth. Stir together.
6. Reduce the heat to low, cover and cook for 25 minutes until the noodles are cooked.
7. Top with parmesan and serve.

Nutrition: Calories: 643 Net carbs: 57g Fat: 23g Protein: 35g

38. Beef and Cheese Gratin

Preparation Time: 5 minutes

Cooking Time: 15 minutes

Servings: 4

Ingredients:

- 1 ½ lb. steak mince
- 2/3 cup beef stock
- 3 oz. Mozzarella or cheddar cheese, grated
- 3 oz. butter, melted
- 7 oz. breadcrumbs
- 1 tablespoon extra-virgin olive oil
- 1 x roast vegetable pack
- 1 x red onion, diced
- 1 x red pepper, diced
- 1 x 14 oz. can chop tomatoes
- 1 x zucchini, diced
- 3 cloves garlic, crushed
- 1 tablespoon Worcestershire sauce
- For the topping…
- Fresh thyme

Directions:

1. Pop a skillet over a medium heat and add the oil.
2. Add the red pepper, onion, zucchini and garlic. Cook for 5 minutes.
3. Add the beef and cook for five minutes.

4. Throw in the tinned tomatoes, beef stock and Worcestershire sauce then stir well.
5. Bring to the boil then simmer for 6 minutes.
6. Divide between the bowls and top with the thyme.
7. Serve and enjoy.

Nutrition: Calories: 678 Net carbs: 24g Fat: 45g Protein: 48g

SIDE DISH AND PIZZA

39. Lemony Barley and Yogurt

Preparation time: 10 minutes

Cooking time: 30 minutes

Servings: 4

Ingredients:

- ½ cup barley
- 1 and ½ cup veggie stock
- ½ cup Greek yogurt
- Salt and black pepper to the taste
- 2 tablespoons olive oil
- 1 tablespoon lemon juice
- ¼ cup mint, chopped
- 1 apple, cored and chopped

Directions:

1. Put barley in a pot, add the stock and salt, bring to a boil and simmer for 30 minutes.
2. Drain, transfer the barley to a bowl, add the rest of the ingredients, toss, divide between plates and serve as a side dish.

Nutrition: calories 263, fat 9, fiber 11.4, carbs 17.4, protein 6.5

40. Chard and Couscous

Preparation time: 10 minutes

Cooking time: 10 minutes

Servings: 4

Ingredients:

- 10 ounces couscous
- 1 and ½ cup hot water
- 2 garlic cloves, minced
- 2 tablespoons olive oil
- ½ cup raisins
- 2 bunches Swiss chard, chopped
- Salt and black pepper to the taste

Directions:

1. Put couscous in a bowl, add the water, stir, cover, leave aside for 10 minutes and fluff with a fork.
2. Heat up a pan with the oil over medium heat, add the garlic, and sauté for 1 minute.
3. Add the couscous and the rest of the ingredients, toss, divide between plates and serve.

Nutrition: calories 300, fat 6.9, fiber 11.4, carbs 17.4, protein 6

41. Chili Cabbage and Coconut

Preparation time: 5 minutes

Cooking time: 20 minutes

Servings: 4

Ingredients:

- 3 tablespoons olive oil
- 1 spring curry leaves, chopped
- 1 teaspoon mustard seeds, crushed
- 1 green cabbage head, shredded
- 4 green chili peppers, chopped
- ½ cup coconut flesh, grated
- Salt and black pepper to the taste

Directions:

1. Heat up a pan with the oil over medium heat, add the curry leaves, mustard seeds and the chili peppers and cook for 5 minutes.
2. Add the rest of the ingredients, toss and cook for 15 minutes more.
3. Divide the mix between plates and serve as a side dish.

Nutrition: calories 221, fat 5.5, fiber 11.1, carbs 22.1, protein 6.7

42. Chickpeas, Figs and Couscous

Preparation time: 10 minutes

Cooking time: 20 minutes

Servings: 4

Ingredients:

1. 1 red onion, chopped
2. 2 tablespoons olive oil
3. 2 garlic cloves, minced
4. 28 ounces canned chickpeas, drained and rinsed
5. 2 cups veggie stock
6. 2 cups couscous, cooked
7. 2 tablespoons coriander, chopped
8. ½ cup figs, dried and chopped
9. Salt and black pepper to the taste

Directions:

1. Heat up a pan with the oil over medium heat, add the onion and the garlic, stir and sauté for 5 minutes.
2. Add the chickpeas and the rest of the ingredients except the couscous and cook over medium heat for 15 minutes stirring often.
3. Divide the couscous between plates, divide the chickpeas mix on top and serve.

Nutrition: calories 263, fat 11.5, fiber 9.45, carbs 22.4, protein 7.3

43. Cheesy Tomato Salad

Preparation time: 5 minutes

Cooking time: 0 minutes

Servings: 4

Ingredients:

- 2 pounds tomatoes, sliced
- 1 red onion, chopped
- Sea salt and black pepper to the taste
- 4 ounces feta cheese, crumbled
- 2 tablespoons mint, chopped
- A drizzle of olive oil

Directions:

1. In a salad bowl, mix the tomatoes with the onion and the rest of the ingredients, toss and serve as a side salad.

Nutrition: calories 190, fat 4.5, fiber 3.4, carbs 8.7, protein 3.3

44. Balsamic Tomato Mix

Preparation time: 6 minutes

Cooking time: 0 minutes

Servings: 4

Ingredients:

- 2 pounds cherry tomatoes, halved
- 2 tablespoons olive oil
- 2 tablespoons balsamic vinegar
- 1 garlic clove, minced
- 1 cup basil, chopped
- 1 tablespoon chives, chopped
- Salt and black pepper to the taste

Directions:

1. In a bowl, combine the tomatoes with the garlic, basil and the rest of the ingredients, toss and serve as a side salad.

Nutrition: calories 200, fat 5.6, fiber 4.5, carbs 15.1, protein 4.3

VEGETARIAN DISHES

45. Steamed Squash Chowder

Preparation Time: 20 minutes

Cooking Time: 40 minutes

Servings: 4

Ingredients:

- 3 cups chicken broth
- 2 tbsp. ghee
- 1 tsp. chili powder
- ½ tsp. cumin
- 1 ½ tsp. salt
- 2 tsp. cinnamon
- 3 tbsp. olive oil
- 2 carrots, chopped
- 1 small yellow onion, chopped
- 1 green apple, sliced and cored
- 1 large butternut squash, peeled, seeded, and chopped to ½-inch cubes

Directions:

2. In a large pot on medium high fire, melt ghee.
3. Once ghee is hot, sauté onions for 5 minutes or until soft and translucent.
4. Add olive oil, chili powder, cumin, salt, and cinnamon. Sauté for half a minute.

5. Add chopped squash and apples.
6. Sauté for 10 minutes while stirring once in a while.
7. Add broth, cover and cook on medium fire for twenty minutes or until apples and squash are tender.
8. With an immersion blender, puree chowder. Adjust consistency by adding more water.
9. Add more salt or pepper depending on desire.
10. Serve and enjoy.

Nutrition: Calories: 228; Carbs: 17.9g; Protein: 2.2g; Fat: 18.0g

46. Steamed Zucchini-Paprika

Preparation Time: 15 minutes

Cooking Time: 30 minutes

Servings: 2

Ingredients:

- 4 tbsp. olive oil
- 3 cloves of garlic, minced
- 1 onion, chopped
- 3 medium-sized zucchinis, sliced thinly
- A dash of paprika
- Salt and pepper to taste

Directions:

1. Place all ingredients in the Instant Pot.
2. Give a good stir to combine all ingredients.
3. Close the lid and make sure that the steam release valve is set to "Venting."
4. Press the "Slow Cook" button and adjust the cooking time to 4 hours.
5. Halfway through the cooking time, open the lid and give a good stir to brown the other side.

Nutrition: Calories: 93; Carbs: 3.1g; Protein: 0.6g; Fat: 10.2g

47. Orange and Cucumber Salad

Preparation Time: 10 minutes

Cooking Time: 0 minutes

Servings: 4

Ingredients:

- 2 cucumbers, sliced
- 1 orange, peeled and cut into segments
- 1 cup cherry tomatoes, halved
- 1 small red onion, chopped
- 3 tbsp. olive oil
- 4 and ½ tsp. balsamic vinegar
- Salt and black pepper to the taste
- 1 tbsp. lemon juice

Directions:

1. In a bowl, mix the cucumbers with the orange and the rest of the ingredients, toss and serve cold.

Nutrition: Calories 102, Fat 7.5g, Fiber 3g, Carbs 6.1g, Protein 3.4g

48. Parsley and Corn Salad

Preparation Time: 10 minutes

Cooking Time: 0 minutes

Servings: 4

Ingredients:

- 1 and ½ tsp. balsamic vinegar
- 2 tbsp. lime juice
- 2 tbsp. olive oil
- A pinch of sea salt and black pepper
- Black pepper to the taste
- 4 cups corn
- ½ cup parsley, chopped
- 2 spring onions, chopped

Directions:

1. In a salad bowl, combine the corn with the onions and the rest of the ingredients, toss and serve cold.

Nutrition: Calories 121, Fat 9.5g, Fiber 1.8g, Carbs 4.1g, Protein 1.9g

FISH AND SEAFOOD

49. Dijon Mustard and Lime Marinated Shrimp

Preparation Time: 10 minutes

Cooking Time: 10 minutes

Servings: 8

Ingredients:

- ½ cup fresh lime juice, plus lime zest as garnish
- ½ cup rice vinegar
- ½ tsp. hot sauce
- 1 bay leaf
- 1 cup water
- 1 lb. uncooked shrimp, peeled and deveined
- 1 medium red onion, chopped
- 2 tbsp. capers
- 2 tbsp. Dijon mustard
- 3 whole cloves

Directions:

1. Mix hot sauce, mustard, capers, lime juice and onion in a shallow baking dish and set aside.
2. Bring to a boil in a large saucepan bay leaf, cloves, vinegar and water.
3. Once boiling, add shrimps and cook for a minute while stirring continuously.

4. Drain shrimps and pour shrimps into onion mixture.
5. For an hour, refrigerate while covered the shrimps.
6. Then serve shrimps cold and garnished with lime zest.

Nutrition: Calories: 232.2; Protein: 17.8g; Fat: 3g; Carbs: 15g

50. Dill Relish on White Sea Bass

Preparation Time: 10 minutes

Cooking Time: 12 minutes

Servings: 4

Ingredients:

- 1 ½ tbsp. chopped white onion
- 1 ½ tsp. chopped fresh dill
- 1 lemon, quartered
- 1 tsp. Dijon mustard
- 1 tsp. lemon juice
- 1 tsp. pickled baby capers, drained
- 4 pieces of 4-oz white sea bass fillets

Directions:

1. Preheat oven to 375°F.
2. Mix lemon juice, mustard, dill, capers and onions in a small bowl.
3. Prepare four aluminum foil squares and place 1 fillet per foil.
4. Squeeze a lemon wedge per fish.
5. Evenly divide into 4 the dill spread and drizzle over fillet.
6. Close the foil over the fish securely and pop in the oven.
7. Bake for 10 to 12 minutes or until fish is cooked through.

8. Remove from foil and transfer to a serving platter, serve and enjoy.

Nutrition: Calories: 115; Protein: 7g; Fat: 1g; Carbs: 12g

51. Garlic Roasted Shrimp with Zucchini Pasta

Preparation Time: 10 minutes

Cooking Time: 10 minutes

Servings: 2

Ingredients:

- 2 medium-sized zucchinis, cut into thin strips or spaghetti noodles
- Salt and pepper to taste
- 1 lemon, zested and juiced
- 2 garlic cloves, minced
- 2 tbsp. ghee, melted
- 2 tbsp. olive oil
- 8 oz. shrimps, cleaned and deveined

Directions:

1. Preheat the oven to 400°F.
2. In a mixing bowl, mix all ingredients except the zucchini noodles. Toss to coat the shrimp.
3. Bake for 10 minutes until the shrimps turn pink.
4. Add the zucchini pasta then toss.

Nutrition: Calories: 299; Fat: 23.2g; Protein: 14.3g; Carbs: 10.9g

APPETIZER AND SNAK RECIPES

52. Greek Fava

Preparation time: 10 minutes

Cooking time: 30 minutes

Servings: 4

INGREDIENTS:

- 2 cups Santorini fava (yellow split peas), rinsed
- 2 medium onions, chopped
- 2 ½ cups water
- 2 cups +2 tablespoons vegetable broth
- 1 teaspoon salt or Himalayan pink salt
- To garnish:
- Lemon juice as required
- Chopped parsley

Directions:

1. Place fava in a large pot. Add onions, broth, water and salt and stir. Place over medium heat. When it begins to boil, reduce the heat and cook until fava is tender.
2. Remove from heat and cool. Blend until creamy. Ladle into small plates. Add lemon juice and stir. Garnish with parsley and serve.

Nutrition: Calories 405 Fat 1 g Carbohydrate 75 g Protein 25 g

53. Hummus, Feta & Bell Pepper Crackers

Preparation time: 10 minutes

Cooking time: 0 minutes

Servings: 2

Ingredients:

- 4 tablespoons hummus
- 2 large whole grain crisp bread
- 4 tablespoons crumbled feta
- 1 small bell pepper, diced

Directions:

1. Top the pieces of crisp bread with hummus. Sprinkle feta cheese and bell peppers and serve.

Nutrition: Calories 136 Fat 7 g Carbohydrate 13 g Protein 6 g

54. Tomato & Basil Bruschetta

Preparation time: 10 minutes

Cooking time: 10 minutes

Servings: 3

Ingredients:

- 3 tomatoes, finely chopped
- 1 clove garlic, minced
- ¼ teaspoon garlic powder (optional)
- A handful basil leaves, coarsely chopped
- Salt to taste
- Pepper to taste
- ½ teaspoon olive oil
- ½ tablespoon balsamic vinegar
- ½ tablespoon butter
- ½ baguette French bread or Italian bread, cut into ½ inch thick slices

Directions:

1. Add tomatoes, garlic and basil in a bowl and toss well. Add salt and pepper. Drizzle oil and vinegar and toss well. Set aside for an hour.
2. Melt the butter and brush it over the baguette slices. Place in an oven and toast the slices. Sprinkle the tomato mixture on top and serve right away.

Nutrition: Calories 162 Fat 4 g Carbohydrate 29 g Protein 4 g

DESSERT RECIPES

55. Wrapped Plums

Preparation Time: 5 minutes

Cooking Time: 0 minutes

Servings: 8

Ingredients:

- 2 ounces prosciutto, cut into 16 pieces
- 4 plums, quartered
- 1 tablespoon chives, chopped
- A pinch of red pepper flakes, crushed

Directions:

1. Wrap each plum quarter in a prosciutto slice, arrange them all on a platter, sprinkle the chives and pepper flakes all over and serve.

Nutrition: Calories 30 Fat 1g Carbohydrates 4g Protein 2g

56. Marinated Feta and Artichokes

Preparation Time: 10 minutes, plus 4 hours inactive time

Cooking Time: 10 minutes

Servings: 2

Ingredients:

- 4 ounces traditional Greek feta, cut into ½-inch cubes
- 4 ounces drained artichoke hearts, quartered lengthwise
- 1/3 cup extra-virgin olive oil
- Zest and juice of 1 lemon
- 2 tablespoons roughly chopped fresh rosemary
- 2 tablespoons roughly chopped fresh parsley
- ½ teaspoon black peppercorns

Directions:

1. In a glass bowl combine the feta and artichoke hearts. Add the olive oil, lemon zest and juice, rosemary, parsley, and peppercorns and toss gently to coat, being sure not to crumble the feta.
2. Cool for 4 hours, or up to 4 days. Take out of the refrigerator 30 minutes before serving.

Nutrition: Calories 235 Fat 23g Carbohydrates 1g Protein 4g

57. Tuna Croquettes

Preparation Time: 40 minutes

Cooking Time: 25 minutes

Servings: 36

Ingredients:

- 6 tablespoons extra-virgin olive oil, plus 1 to 2 cups
- 5 tablespoons almond flour, plus 1 cup, divided
- 1¼ cups heavy cream
- 1 (4-ounce) can olive oil-packed yellowfin tuna
- 1 tablespoon chopped red onion
- 2 teaspoons minced capers
- ½ teaspoon dried dill
- ¼ teaspoon freshly ground black pepper
- 2 large eggs
- 1 cup panko breadcrumbs (or a gluten-free version)

Directions:

1. In a large skillet, warm up 6 tablespoons olive oil over medium-low heat. Add 5 tablespoons almond flour and cook, stirring constantly, until a smooth paste forms and the flour browns slightly, 2 to 3 minutes.

2. Select the heat to medium-high and gradually mix in the heavy cream, whisking constantly until completely smooth and thickened, another 4 to 5 minutes. Remove and add in the tuna, red onion, capers, dill, and pepper.

3. Transfer the mixture to an 8-inch square baking dish that is well coated with olive oil and set aside at room temperature.

4. Wrap and cool for 4 hours or up to overnight. To form the croquettes, set out three bowls. In one, beat together the eggs.

5. In another, add the remaining almond flour. In the third, add the panko. Line a baking sheet with parchment paper.

6. Scoop about a tablespoon of cold prepared dough into the flour mixture and roll to coat. Shake off excess and, using your hands, roll into an oval.

7. Dip the croquette into the beaten egg, then lightly coat in panko. Set on lined baking sheet and repeat with the remaining dough.

8. In a small saucepan, warm up the remaining 1 to 2 cups of olive oil, over medium-high heat.

9. Once the oil is heated, fry the croquettes 3 or 4 at a time, depending on the size of your pan, removing with a slotted spoon when golden brown.

10. You will need to adjust the temperature of the oil occasionally to prevent burning. If the croquettes get dark brown very quickly, lower the temperature.

Nutrition: Calories 245 Fat 22g Carbohydrates 1g Protein 6g

58. Smoked Salmon Crudités

Preparation Time: 10 minutes

Cooking Time: 15 minutes

Servings: 4

Ingredients:

- 6 ounces smoked wild salmon
- 2 tablespoons Roasted Garlic Aioli
- 1 tablespoon Dijon mustard
- 1 tablespoon chopped scallions, green parts only
- 2 teaspoons chopped capers
- ½ teaspoon dried dill
- 4 endive spears or hearts of romaine
- ½ English cucumber, cut into ¼-inch-thick rounds

Directions:

1. Roughly cut the smoked salmon and transfer in a small bowl. Add the aioli, Dijon, scallions, capers, and dill and mix well.
2. Top endive spears and cucumber rounds with a spoonful of smoked salmon mixture and enjoy chilled.

Nutrition: Calories 92 Fat 5g Carbohydrates 1g Protein 9g

59. Citrus-Marinated Olives

Preparation Time: 4 hours

Cooking Time: 0 minutes

Servings: 2

Ingredients:

- 2 cups mixed green olives with pits
- ¼ cup red wine vinegar
- ¼ cup extra-virgin olive oil
- 4 garlic cloves, finely minced
- Zest and juice of 1 large orange
- 1 teaspoon red pepper flakes
- 2 bay leaves
- ½ teaspoon ground cumin
- ½ teaspoon ground allspice

Directions:

1. Incorporate the olives, vinegar, oil, garlic, orange zest and juice, red pepper flakes, bay leaves, cumin, and allspice and mix well.
2. Seal and chill for 4 hours or up to a week to allow the olives to marinate, tossing again before serving.

Nutrition: Calories 133 Fat 14g Carbohydrates 2g Protein 1g

60. Olive Tapenade with Anchovies

Preparation Time: 1hour and 10 minutes

Cooking Time: 0 minutes

Servings: 2

Ingredients:

- 2 cups pitted Kalamata olives or other black olives
- 2 anchovy fillets, chopped
- 2 teaspoons chopped capers
- 1 garlic clove, finely minced
- 1 cooked egg yolk
- 1 teaspoon Dijon mustard
- ¼ cup extra-virgin olive oil
- Seedy Crackers, Versatile Sandwich Round, or vegetables, for serving (optional)

Directions:

1. Rinse the olives in cold water and drain well. In a food processor, blender, or a large jar (if using an immersion blender) place the drained olives, anchovies, capers, garlic, egg yolk, and Dijon.
2. Process until it forms a thick paste. While running, gradually stream in the olive oil. Handover to a small bowl, cover, and refrigerate at least 1 hour to let the flavors develop.
3. Serve with Seedy Crackers, atop a Versatile Sandwich Round, or with your favorite crunchy vegetables.

Nutrition: Calories 179 Fat 19g Carbohydrates 2g Protein 2g

.

Lightning Source UK Ltd.
Milton Keynes UK
UKHW021833040621
384966UK00002B/461